Lifestyle

First Aid

9 Simple Concepts to Supercharge

Your Health and Your Life

**Also by Andre Panagos M.D.
and Marwa Ahmed M.D.**
Your Top Back Pain Questions Answered

Also by Andre Panagos M.D.
Spine: Rehabilitation Medicine Quick Reference Series

Lifestyle
First Aid

9 Simple Concepts to Supercharge

Your Health and Your Life

Marwa Ahmed, M.D., M.S.

Andre Panagos, M.D., M.Sc.

Second Avenue Press

New York, NY

SECOND AVENUE PRESS
Lifestyle First Aid, 9 Simple Concepts to Supercharge Your Health and Your Life
Marwa Ahmed, Andre Panagos

Printed in the United States of America by Second Avenue Press

10 9 8 7 6 5 4 3 2 1

Contents

Preface

Every single day our patients ask us how they can permanently treat their chronic back pain, sports and musculoskeletal injuries. In the past, we have answered with the same phrase you may have heard many times before, "Eat right, exercise, and get plenty of rest." A growing body of scientific research continues to demonstrate its importance, yet it is nearly impossible to do this in our modern world. What is even more surprising is that many of us have forgotten how to eat nutritious meals, incorporate daily exercise into our schedule, and get a good night's sleep. The outcome of all of these poor habits is that we develop chronic ailments such as arthritis, muscle deconditioning, chronic pain, anxiety, and depression which bring our lives to a screeching halt.

We combed through volumes of medical research and found a surprising amount of overlooked information pertaining to healing and tissue regeneration. We have highlighted the main points in this book which has resulted in amazing successes for our patients, ourselves and our loved ones. In many cases, we have saved people from a downward spiral of declining health and years of grotesque pain and disability. We believe this information will have a profound impact in your ability to heal and thrive in our modern world. This will make you healthier than you ever thought possible. We are excited to share this book with you to re-introduce simple concepts to eat right, exercise and get adequate sleep, as well as other secrets to supercharge your life every single day.

To your health,

Marwa Ahmed, M.D. and Andre Panagos M.D.
New York, NY
February, 2015

Chapter 1

A Perspective on the Fundamental Anti-Inflammatory Diet

"Let food be thy medicine and medicine be thy food."
Hippocrates

What is an anti-inflammatory diet?
An anti-inflammatory diet is one in which fresh fruits, vegetables, meat and seafood are eaten with little or no intake of processed foods. The purpose of this style of eating is to eat foods that are high in vitamins and minerals along with healthy proteins and fats to support the growth and repair of your body.

Why is an anti-inflammatory diet important?
Now more than ever, our society is plagued by a wide variety of chronic diseases. And while it may not be accepted by mainstream society, it has everything to do with your diet. Scientific research and clinical experience have shown that dietary modifications

and administration of nutrients and other natural substances are frequently and almost consistently effective for both preventing and treating a wide range of symptoms and illnesses.

Over the past several generations, we have established a new standard diet of highly processed foods that are high in sugar and fat and low in fiber. Furthermore, modern farming techniques are designed to produce high crop yields at the expense of low nutrient density. As a result, we consume more calories

Our diets have drastically changed over the past 50-100 years.

with fewer vitamins and micronutrients than our ancestors did. Many experts believe this is a major cause of chronic diseases such as heart disease, cancer and chronic pain.

Why is sugar such a problem?
The average American consumes 44 teaspoons of sugar per day. Sugar is used to mask inferior ingredients in products, improve flavor, and has over 50 different aliases in the list of ingredients such as high-fructose corn syrup, dextrose, rice syrup, mannitol and evaporated cane juice. Sugar is one of the most dangerous and addictive substances in our diet. Research studies have shown sugar to be more addictive than alcohol, cocaine and even heroin. Artificial sweeteners such as Aspartame (NutraSweet®) breakdown to components that are known to be neurotoxic. We all know that excessive sugar consumption contributes to obesity and tooth decay but it also contributes to the development of other symptoms and diseases including chronic

Sugar, flour and dairy products promote inflammation, so they basically contribute to sickness and disease.

pain, fatigue, anxiety, migraine headaches, high cholesterol, liver disease, osteoporosis, hypertension, diabetes mellitus, cancer and heart disease.

What is wrong with bread?
We cannot tell you how often we hear our patients tell us, "I love bread and I can't live without it" and we understand, as it is a staple in cuisines around the world. Over the past 50 years however, wheat

has undergone a dramatic and drastic makeover. Hybridization and genetic manipulation by agricultural scientists focused on increasing yield have turned modern wheat into a distant relative of the grain our ancestors once consumed. The current strains of wheat that are available today are so unique that they are unable to survive in the wild without human support and many scientists also believe that wheat has begun to interfere with our immune systems.

The nutrient-rich germ portion and the nutrient and fiber-rich bran portion of grain is removed during the milling process. As a result, ingesting these processed grains impairs your body's ability to control blood sugar. Flour contains substantially lower amounts of vitamins, minerals, and fiber than in the past. Your body treats the small flour molecules like sugar with the same risk of developing the diseases mentioned earlier. This is independent of the gluten molecule that many people with celiac disease are allergic to, which creates its own havoc within the gastrointestinal system.

Extruded grains such as breakfast cereal, as well as puffed wheat, puffed oats and puffed rice are processed using high heat and pressure which makes them virtually indigestible. This creates a food that is even worse for your body than sugar. It is no wonder that breakfast cereals are fortified with vitamins and minerals.

Sprouted whole grains, however, unlock the essential vitamins and nutrients that are naturally present within the grain. Sprouting neutralizes phytic acid, which is known to block the absorption of nutrients by the intestinal track, as well as a number of other enzyme inhibitors making this form of grain more nutritious.

Does milk really do a body good?

Research has demonstrated that cow's milk is one of the most common food allergens in the American diet. From an evolutionary perspective, your body may be able to digest milk, but pasteurized and homogenized milk as well as the various low-fat and non-fat milk products involve a great deal of processing, which ultimately makes them more difficult to digest. Recent research has demonstrated that milk does not offer any nutrients including calcium, proteins and fats that cannot be found in other healthier animal or whole plant foods. Contrary to popular belief:

- You can get much more vitamin D from just a few minutes of direct sun exposure than from milk. Research suggests vitamin D is more important than calcium for bone health.

- Milk products have never been shown to reduce fracture risk and may also increase your risk of death due to the high quantity of natural sugar (lactose) found in milk (Michaëlsson K et. al 2014).

If I keep eating these foods, what can happen?

The side effects of a nutrient-deficient diet are more profound than you have probably ever imagined. Foods that are unhealthy are the exact ones that are subsidized by the government, so they are made more affordable, which promotes a vicious cycle of greater consumption and illness. Consuming disease-promoting, nutrient-deficient foods over decades not only reduces your intake of vital nutrients, but also increases the burden on your body, speeding up the depletion of nutrients from your body. A new field of nutritional genomics is beginning to unlock the secrets of the effects of food and nutrition on your DNA. Scientists can now study how food and nutrients change the way your cells use your DNA code and the proteins made from it. If the cells are not working optimally, this sets the stage for a variety of illnesses mentioned previously, as well as mitochondrial dysfunction believed to be involved in the onset of cancer, inflammatory and autoimmune diseases. It is not a question of if, but rather when a disease will interrupt your busy lifestyle.

> **Americans are leading lives of hidden hunger in an "overnourished" but "nutrient deficient" society.**

What are some easy things I can do to improve my diet?

You can start by eliminating or significantly reducing your daily intake of sugar, flour and dairy products and increasing your intake of fresh, local vegetables and healthy proteins every day. Michael Pollan, the author of numerous books on food including, "The Omnivore's Dilemma" and "In Defense of Food," believes you should eat local food closest to its natural state. While changing one's dietary habits is no easy task, you will begin to see changes within three to six months. Our patients have reported improved sleep, greater energy and focus, as well as improved vision, stronger hair and nails, and better looking skin. We are especially excited to hear patients report that they have discontinued blood pressure, cholesterol, diabetes, anti-depressant and reflux medications as a result of these dietary changes. Once you start feeling better it is very hard to return to your old diet.

To get you started with your new dietary habits, make sure you include proteins, healthy fats, vegetables and fruits with each meal to feel satiated. Remember to:

- Eat a colorful variety of local vegetables more often than fruits.
- Get to know the vendors at the local farmer's market and buy foods that are in season to maximize their nutrient content.
- Cook your own food, as restaurants focus on flavor, not health.
- Exclude or greatly minimize your consumption of prepared and processed foods from crinkly bags, boxes, containers and cans.
- Snack on raw or sprouted nuts, seeds, raw vegetables or some fruit between meals if needed.
- Become an expert label reader and learn more about the scientific ingredients in food. Generally, if you cannot pronounce it, you should not eat it.
- Take time to chew and digest your food and do not eat while walking since poor digestion equals starvation.
- Sit down and enjoy your food with family and friends.

Ideas for Promoting an Anti-Inflammatory Diet

Type of Food	Nutrient Value	Recommendations
Vegetables and Fruit	Fruits and vegetables are rich sources of vitamins, minerals, carotenoids, flavinoids, fiber, and phytochemicals.	Eat abundant amounts of vegetables daily in all colors of the rainbow. Eat fruit daily but in moderation due to their natural sugar (fructose) content, in all colors of the rainbow.
Protein	Protein from grass-fed, hormone-free, antibiotic-free and non-GMO sources are ideal and are good sources of protein as well as omega-3 fatty acids and other nutrients.	Eat animal protein including beef, lamb, poultry, eggs, organ meats and homemade gelatin-rich bone broth. Eat small, wild fish and shellfish. Choose wisely as our oceans are over-fished and polluted.

Grains	Sprouted whole grains are a good source of vitamins and minerals.	Eat sprouted whole grains that have not been highly processed such as bulgar, spelt, kamut, buckwheat, oats, farro and brown rice.
Dairy	Dairy can be a rich source of nutrients.	Butter, cheese, yoghurt and other whole milk products derived from grass-fed animals are very healthy. Consider sheep or goat milk products over cow milk if available. Remove or limit consumption of pasteurized and homogenized milk in addition to skim, low-fat and non-fat milk, cheese and yoghurt products.
Sugar	No nutritional value	Reduce or eliminate intake of all sugar products including cereal, granola and energy bars, fruit yoghurt and candy. Avoid high-fructose corn syrup. Remove artificial sweeteners as they are more toxic than sugar.
Oils	Good source of important fatty acids	Extra virgin olive oil is safe to use in it's natural state on salads or in low heat applications. Coconut oil is better suited for high heat applications. Remove all vegetable oils and canola oil as their production makes them pro-inflammatory.
Beverages	Essential for keeping hydrated, flushing out toxins from your body and can be a source of antioxidants	Replace regular and diet soda, fruit juices and sugary iced tea with water, lemon water or dilute tea. Drink more tea and less coffee as it has lower levels of caffeine and is a great source of antioxidants.

Resources:

1. Davis, William. Wheat Belly: Lose the Wheat, Lose the Weight, and Find Your Path Back to Health. Emmaus, Penn.: Rodale, 2011. Print.
2. Gaby, Alan. "A Review of the Fundamentals of Diet." Global Advances in Health and Medicine 2.1 (2013): 58-63. Print
3. "Got Proof? Lack of Evidence for Milk's Benefits - Dr. Mark Hyman." Dr Mark Hyman. 05 July 2013. Web. 16 Jan. 2015. <http://drhyman.com/blog/2013/07/05/got-proof-lack-of-evidence-for-milks-benefits/>.
4. "Lactose Intolerance." Genetics Home Reference. Web. 15 Jan. 2015. <http://ghr.nlm.nih.gov/condition/lactose-intolerance>.
5. Michaëlsson K, Wolk A, Langenskiöld S, Basu S, Warensjö Lemming E, Melhus H, Byberg L. Milk intake and risk of mortality and fractures in women and men: cohort studies. BMJ. 2014 Oct 28;349:g6015. Print.
6. Sales, N. M. R., P. B. Pelegrini, and M. C. Goersch. "Nutrigenomics: Definitions and Advances of This New Science." Journal of Nutrition and Metabolism 2014 (2014): 1-6. Print.

Chapter 2

A Magnesium Scarcity Paradox that is More Colossal than Ever

What is magnesium?
Magnesium is a mineral found in the earth's crust that is essential to all living cells and is very important for your health.

What is the role of magnesium and why is it so important?
Magnesium is the most overlooked mineral on earth. It is involved in over 350 different biochemical reactions and functions in the body, including muscle and nerve function, blood pressure, glucose control, energy production and bone health.

Where can magnesium be found?
Magnesium is found in the earth's crust so it dissolves in water, making it widely distributed in plant and animal foods. Rivers, streams and well water all have magnesium dissolved within it, but municipal water systems condition the water to limit corrosion of pipes. This can greatly reduce the amount of magnesium dissolved in the water you use at the tap. The magnesium content in bottled

water varies greatly depending on the source and processing of the water.

Why am I magnesium deficient?
The scarcity paradox is that despite widespread distribution of magnesium, an amazing 75% of the population is deficient due to various dietary, environmental, and drug-related factors. As a result, it has become increasingly difficult to meet your daily requirements through your diet alone.

Causes of Low Magnesium Intake

Low Bioavailability	Only 30-40% of dietary magnesium consumed is actually absorbed by the body.
Processed Foods, Soda, Drugs, Caffeine and Alcohol	Magnesium is flushed from the system with consumption of processed foods and drugs.
Water Purification	Modern water treatment processes have depleted municipal water of magnesium.
Modern Agriculture	Modern farming relies heavily on the use of chemical fertilizers and pesticides which have heavily depleted the earth's topsoil of their mineral content.
Chronic Stress	Physical and emotional stress is associated with greater magnesium utilization by the body.

What are the dangers of magnesium deficiency?
Low intake of magnesium over time can increase the risk of illness:

Early signs	As the deficiency worsens	Severe deficiency
Loss of appetite Nausea/Vomiting Dizziness Fatigue and weakness	Acute and chronic migraine headaches Numbness and tingling Muscle twitching, cramps, spasms and tremors Seizures, poor memory, anxiety, and insomnia	Disruption of mineral homeostasis Osteoporosis Diabetes mellitus

What should my magnesium level be?
We routinely test for red blood cell (RBC) magnesium. A reference range of 4.2-6.8 milligrams per deciliter (mg/dL) is considered normal; that is, normal for our "sick" population. We have noticed significant improvement in patients by targeting a value of at least 6 mg/dL.

What are great sources of magnesium rich foods?

There are many foods that have a great amount of magnesium. Try to incorporate the following foods into your diet:

- Dark green leafy vegetables such as spinach, kale and collard greens
- Avocados
- Legumes
- Nuts and seeds such as squash and pumpkin seeds, brazil nuts, almonds and cashews
- Bananas
- Dried fruit such as figs and dates
- Whole grains such as brown rice and buckwheat
- Dark chocolate
- Mineral water- but you need to check the label to be sure there is magnesium in it

What should I do to get adequate magnesium in my diet?

While meeting your daily magnesium requirements through diet would be ideal, this has become increasingly difficult as mentioned previously. Thus, supplementation plays an important role and is considered a safe, effective way to ensure adequate magnesium intake.

We cannot tell you how many of our patients have had remarkable improvement. The recommended dietary allowances (RDAs) based on government calculations are based on estimates that are known to be well below optimum levels. RDAs are simply not designed to address the possibility that higher levels of nutrient intake can help treat and prevent chronic diseases as well as enhance overall well-being. RDAs for magnesium range from 80-420 mg, based on age and gender. Magnesium supplements are available in a variety of forms and not all are created equal. Magnesium applied to the skin can be absorbed directly into your cells, bypassing the digestive system. This may be a convenient solution for those unable to tolerate oral magnesium due to diarrhea.

Recommended Oral Formulations[1]	Recommended Transdermal Formulations
Magnesium Citrate/Gluconate Magnesium Glycinate/Lysinate/Taurate Magnesium Chloride/Sulfate	Magnesium Oil Magnesium Lotion Epsom Salts (1-2 cups in a hot bath for 20-30 minutes)[2]

[1] Avoid magnesium oxide as it has poor bioavailability
[2] As a caution, rise from your bath slowly and carefully as the hot water and steam can precipitate dizziness

What supplement dose should I take?

We recommend that adults start with either 400-600 mg total per day (not to exceed 800 mg total per day) in divided doses with meals. If there is no or little noticeable improvement in symptoms or overall well-being, slowly titrate up towards the maximum dosage as directed by your physician. Ultimately, you will be limited in how far you can titrate up as there is a bowel tolerance threshold that brings on stomach irritation, loose stool or diarrhea if exceeded. This is the reason why magnesium is the primary ingredient in some laxatives.

Resources:

1. Calcium and Magnesium in Drinking-water: Public Health Significance. Geneva, Switzerland: World Health Organization, 2009. Print.
2. Gaby, Alan. "A Review of the Fundamentals of Diet." Global Advances in Health and Medicine 2.1 (2013): 58-63. Print.
3. "Magnesium." — Health Professional Fact Sheet. Web. 18 Jan. 2015. <http://ods.od.nih.gov/factsheets/Magnesium-HealthProfessional/>.
4. "Magnesium Supplementation." Magnesium Supplements & Types of Magnesium. Web. 18 Jan. 2015. <http://www.ancient-minerals.com/magnesium-supplements/>.
5. Calcium and Magnesium in Drinking-water: Public Health Significance. Geneva, Switzerland: World Health Organization, 2009. Print.

Chapter 3

The Fascinating and Simple Truth about Vitamin D

What is vitamin D?
Vitamin D is a fat-soluble pre-hormone that is primarily made following sun exposure on your skin. It can also be found in some foods, although it is thought that sun exposure is the best way to absorb vitamin D.

What is the role of vitamin D and why is it so important?
Until just a few years ago, vitamin D was simply known as the "bone vitamin." Recently research has found that it is used in virtually every single cell in the body and we now appreciate its greater spectrum of importance. There is compelling evidence for its vital role in a tremendous number of physiologic functions such as immune function, mineral homeostasis, cardiovascular function, and neurological function. Vitamin D also regulates genes that control cell growth and development and may be important in cancer prevention.

How widespread is vitamin D deficiency?

It is estimated that one billion people worldwide are vitamin D deficient and at least 64% of Americans do not have enough vitamin D which is thought to increase the risk of chronic disease. Deficiency has even been found in desert areas of the world such as the Middle East due to traditional clothing styles and time spent indoors.

Where can vitamin D be found?

Unlike other vitamins which are typically obtained from your diet, the vast majority of the vitamin D your body utilizes is synthesized directly from UVB exposure from the sun, hence its nickname, "the sunshine vitamin". Vitamin D can also be found in some foods, although vitamin D synthesized from the sun is considered a superior form.

How can I get more vitamin D in my diet?

Some great sources of dietary vitamin D include:

- Cod liver oil and oily fish such as salmon and mackerel
- Organ meats from organically raised, grass-fed animals
- Portobello mushrooms

What are the dangers of vitamin D deficiency?

Nowadays, it is clear that maintaining less than optimal levels of vitamin D can be catastrophic. It opens the door to a host of diseases spanning all organ systems of the body, from cardiovascular disease, diabetes, osteoporosis, dementia to musculoskeletal pain, weakness, inflammatory disorders, cancer, immune dysfunction and autoimmune disorders. Without adequate vitamin D, your tissues cannot operate at their peak capacity so some functions suffer, while others outright fail.

Emerging research suggests that blood levels of vitamin D are a good barometer of overall health.

What should my vitamin D level be?

Checking individual vitamin D blood levels is still not standard of care for many physicians, but it is one of the most important health-protecting steps you can take. Vitamin D deficiency requires immediate attention and aggressive vitamin D replacement.

Understanding Your Vitamin D Level

Deficient Blood Levels	Insufficient Blood Levels	Sufficient Blood Levels	Optimal Blood Levels	Toxic Blood Levels
< or = to 20 ng/mL	21-29 ng/mL	At least 30 ng/mL	50-80 ng/mL	> 100 ng/mL

What are risk factors for vitamin D deficiency?

1. **Aging**: As we get older, our skin changes which leads to a decreased capacity to synthesize vitamin D in the skin when exposed to the sun's UVB light rays.
2. **Sunscreen and Clothing**: Sunscreen and clothing material are effective barriers in blocking the sun's rays necessary for vitamin D formation. The proper application of sunscreen with an SPF factor as low as SPF-15 absorbs 99% of UVB rays, reducing the production of vitamin D by 99% (Holick M, et. al. 2008).
3. **Dark-Skin**: The pigment in our skin called melanin, is a natural and protective sunscreen and is present in greater quantities the darker your skin. This requires more sun exposure to maintain adequate vitamin D levels.
4. **Latitude**: The earth's ozone layer absorbs a portion of the sun's UVB radiation. The further you live from the equator, the greater the distance the sun's rays have to travel and the less UVB radiation reaches your skin.
5. **Obesity**: Vitamin D gets deposited and sequestered in body fat stores making it less bioavailable for your body's tissues.
6. **Inflammatory Bowel Disease and Fat Malabsorption Syndromes**: An unhealthy gastrointestinal system impairs absorption of vitamin D ingested from foods.

What should I do to maintain my vitamin D levels?

There are three routes by which you can successfully correct your vitamin D levels. As with any nutritional deficiency, it is ideal to correct it first through natural means so start by having more fun in the sun!

Ways to Increase Vitamin D Levels

Increase sun exposure	It is possible to obtain your entire vitamin D requirement via sunlight exposure. Aim for 15-30 minutes of direct sun exposure (arms/legs +/- torso). If you expect to be in the sun for a prolonged period of time, set aside some time in the sun before lathering on the sunscreen. *But by all means, protect your face with sunscreen at all times and save yourself the wrinkles!*
Increase dietary intake of vitamin D-rich foods	Very few foods naturally contain vitamin D therefore it is important to recognize that it is essentially impossible to satisfy the body's requirement via dietary sources alone, unless you eat oily fish 3-5 times a week.
Direct ingestion of a vitamin D supplement	The dosage of supplementation[1] depends on your current vitamin D status. Start by having your physician check your vitamin D level via a simple blood test before you take a supplement.

[1]Always balance efforts to improve your vitamin D status with adequate calcium intake.

Resources:

1. Holick, Michael F. "Vitamin D: A D-Lightful Health Perspective." Nutrition Reviews 66 (2008): S182-194. Print.
2. Holick MF. Vitamin D: importance in the prevention of cancers, type 1 diabetes, heart disease, and osteoporosis. Am J Clin Nutr. 79(3) (2004): 362-371. Print
3. Holick, Michael F. "Vitamin D: The Underappreciated D-lightful Hormone That Is Important for Skeletal and Cellular Health." Current Opinion in Endocrinology & Diabetes 9.1 (2002): 87-98. Print.
4. Matsuoka, L. Y., L. Ide, J. Wortsman, J. A. Maclaughlin, and M. F. Holick. "Sunscreens Suppress Cutaneous Vitamin D3 Synthesis." Journal of Clinical Endocrinology & Metabolism 64.6 (1987): 1165-168. Print.
5. Zhang, Ran, and Declan P. Naughton. "Vitamin D in Health and Disease: Current Perspectives." Nutrition Journal 9.1 (2010): 65. Print.

Chapter 4

The Bottom Line on Successful Omega-6 and Omega-3 Fatty Acid Balance

What are fatty acids?

Fatty acids, more commonly referred to as "fats", are macro nutrients that have an effect on cell membrane flexibility and receptor sensitivity, modulate gene expression and serve as precursors of hormone-like compounds called prostaglandins and pro-inflammatory compounds called leukotrienes. They are divided into three general categories.

The Three Types of "Fat"

Saturated Fat	Solid at room temperature. Found in high proportions in animal fat products such as dairy, chocolate, meat and poultry skin. It is also found in tropical oils such as coconut and palm oils.
Monounsaturated Fat	Liquid at room temperature. Most are in the form of omega-9 fatty acids. Found in avocados, canola oil, olive oil, seeds and nuts.

Polyunsaturated Fat	Liquid in room temperature. Subdivided into omega-3 and omega-6 fatty acids. Dietary sources include flax seed, hemp seed, purslane, walnuts and fatty fish.

What are essential fatty acids?

Your body can synthesize all but two of the fats it needs from your diet. Linole**ic** and Linole**nic** acids are the two fatty acids essential to your health that your body cannot make, so they must be obtained directly from foods or purified supplements. These are referred to as essential fatty acids and they are the parent compounds of many omega-6 and omega-3 fatty acids, respectively.

What are omega-6 fatty acids?

Omega-6 fatty acids are polyunsaturated essential fatty acids that are derived from linole**ic** acid. These fats are found in seeds, nuts, grains, dairy, grain-fed livestock and vegetable oils (corn, safflower, soybean, cottonseed, sesame, sunflower). Omega-6 fatty acids are abundant in the standard western diet due to their stability and long shelf life so they are the primary fat found in processed foods. They are the precursors of pro-inflammatory compounds.

What are omega-3 fatty acids?

Omega-3 fatty acids are polyunsaturated essential fatty acids that are derived from linole**nic** acid. The three fatty acid derivatives involved in human physiology are alpha-linolenic acid (ALA), eicosapentaenoic acid (EPA), and docosahexaenoic acid (DHA). They are plentiful in unprocessed foods, fatty fish and in the meat of grass-fed livestock. Omega-3 fatty acids act as anti-inflammatory agents.

What is the role of omega-6 fatty acids and why are they so important?

Not all omega-6 fatty acids behave the same. Most of the omega-6 fatty acids consumed in the standard western diet promote inflammation. Inflammation is often thought of as a bad thing, however it is an important part of your immune system's complex and protective response against harmful viruses and bacteria.

What is the role of omega-3 fatty acids and why are they so important?

Omega-3 fatty acids have anti-inflammatory properties. They have been shown to be beneficial for the prevention and treatment of a wide range of illnesses including cardiovascular disease, stroke, diabetes, autoimmune disorders and cancer.

What are the dangers of omega-3 fatty acid deficiency?

An omega-3 fatty acid deficiency (as well as omega-6 fatty acid deficiency) can lead to a host of symptoms and disorders including joint pain, dry skin, brittle nails and hair, fatigue, mood changes, organ damage and impaired immune function.

What should my Omega-6 and Omega-3 fatty acid levels be?

This is a tricky question because it is not the level of omega-3 fatty acids that matters, but rather the ratio and balance of omega-6 to omega-3 fatty acids. The ideal ratio should be between 1-4:1 (omega-6:omega-3). Unfortunately, the standard American diet has a ratio of omega-6:omega-3 between 10:1 and 25:1. The average intake of omega-3 fatty acids has decreased to less than 20% of what it was 150 years ago. About 95-99% of the population gets omega-3 fatty acids at a level that is less than that required for good health (Kaur N, et. al. 2014). Diets too high in pro-inflammatory omega-6 fatty acids and too low in anti-inflammatory omega-3 fatty acids lead to chronic inflammation, hypertension, and the promotion of blood clots. This increases the risk of serious medical conditions such as heart attack, stroke, inflammatory and autoimmune disorders as well as cancer.

How can I maintain a healthy balance of omega-6 to omega-3 fatty acids?

As with any nutritional deficiency, it is important to correct it through diet. It is possible to obtain your entire omega-3 and omega-6 requirements from diet alone without supplementation. But as the standard American diet is abundant in omega-6 fatty acids, one should simultaneously also focus on limiting processed foods, vegetable oils and conventional grain-fed livestock while improving omega-3 fatty acid intake.

Excellent Sources of Omega-3 Fatty Acids

Dietary sources	Fatty fish (i.e. salmon, mackerel, sardines, herring) Meat (100% grass-fed and pasture-raised beef and chicken) Certain nuts and seeds (i.e. flaxseeds, chia seeds, walnuts) Certain vegetables (i.e. soybeans, brussels sprouts, cauliflower, kale, spinach) Switching to a Mediterranean diet
Supplements	Remember to discuss appropriate dosing with your physician. In general, 2,000-3,000 milligrams of total omega-3 fatty acids taken twice daily with food can be helpful.

It is important to keep in mind that when discussing one nutrient, you cannot ignore others as they are all connected in ways we still do not fully understand. Make sure you have adequate magnesium, zinc, vitamin C and the B vitamins in your diet to ensure that your body will properly utilize the essential fatty acids.

Resources:

1. Gaby, Alan. "A Review of the Fundamentals of Diet." Global Advances in Health and Medicine 2.1 (2013): 58-63. Print.
2. "Gamma-linolenic Acid." University of Maryland Medical Center. Web. 18 Jan. 2015. <http://umm.edu/health/medical/altmed/supplement/gammalinolenic-acid#ixzz3JdSfuETk>.
3. Kaur, Narinder et al. Essential Fatty Acids as Functional Components of Foods - A Review. J Food Sci Technol (October 2014). 51(10):2289-2303.
4. Vasquez Alex. Integrative Orthopedics. Portland,OR: Integrative and Biological Medicine Research and Consulting, 2012, Print.

Chapter 5

Powerful Exercise and Stretching Ideas

"We don't stop playing because we grow old; we grow old because we stop playing."
George Bernard Shaw
(Irish playwright, Nobel prize in Literature)

How can exercise improve my health?

If exercise was a pill it would be a guaranteed best seller with few side effects. We know that exercise has multiple health benefits and plays an important role in successful aging. Some of the many benefits of exercise are that it will:

- Optimize cardiovascular function by strengthening heart muscle
- Raise levels of "good cholesterol" (HDL) and lower levels of "bad cholesterol" (LDL)
- Promote bone health and combat osteoarthritis by improving joint mobility and muscle strength

- Strengthen the immune system
- Improve cognitive function, sleep and decrease anxiety and depression

How much exercise do I need?
Aim for at least 2.5 hours of moderate exercise (where you can talk but do not have the breath to sing) per week. This translates into about 20-30 minutes, 5-7 days per week. Be sure to incorporate interval training which stresses and hence builds muscles more effectively. Always start slow and gradually build up your exercise routine to minimize the risk of injury. If you are older or have a serious medical condition, remember to consult your physician before starting any exercise regimen.

What is the least amount of exercise I can do to get significant health benefits?
The amount of exercise you need for health benefits is much less than you may think. A large study on exercise and mortality found something researchers did not expect, that running for as little as five minutes a day could significantly lower your risk of premature death (Lee D.C. et. al., 2014). So no matter how busy you are, we are sure you can fit in five minutes a day of vigorous exercise, such as running, jump-roping or pedaling vigorously on a stationary bike. Consider simple things in your daily routine such as running for the bus or walking up several flights of stairs while at work. Over the long-term even brief amounts of exercise may add years to your life.

Exercise and stretch daily to lengthen your muscles and possibly your lifespan.

A single session of simple static stretching can result in short-term cardiovascular benefits as well. When you stretch, your brain releases compounds that not only relax your skeletal muscles but also relax the small muscles in the walls of your blood vessels (Farinatti et al., 2011). This results in their dilation, which can lower your blood pressure.

Flexibility on the outside equals healthy flexibility on the inside.

Resources:

1. Brukner, Peter, Karim Khan, and Peter Brukner. Brukner & Khan's Clinical Sports Medicine. Sydney: McGraw-Hill, 2012. Print.
1. Farinatti, Paulo Tv, Carolina Brandão, Pedro Ps Soares, and Antonio Fa Duarte. "Acute Effects of Stretching Exercise on the Heart Rate Variability in Subjects With Low Flexibility Levels." Journal of Strength and Conditioning Research 25.6 (2011): 1579-585. Print.
1. Lee DC, Pate RR, Lavie CJ, Sui X, Church TS, Blair SN. Leisure-Time Running Reduces All-Cause and Cardiovascular Mortality Risk. Journal of the American College of Cardiology, 2014; 64 (5): 472-481. Print.

Chapter 6

The Value of an Uninterrupted Good Night's Sleep

"Dreaming permits each and every one of us to be quietly and
safely insane every night."
Charles A. Fisher

What is sleep?
Sleep is a naturally recurring state characterized by altered consciousness, muscle and sensory activity and waste removal. It is a time of complex neurobiological rejuvenation and growth and appears to be universally vital to life throughout the animal kingdom.

What is the role of sleep and why is it so important?
We spend about one third of our lives sleeping and despite our limited understanding of the purpose and mechanism of sleep, we know that like food, water and oxygen, it is critical for life. Sleep plays a vital role in many body functions including immune regulation, metabolism, tissue repair, learning and memory.

What are the dangers of chronic sleep deprivation?
Sleep deprivation contributes to a wide variety of side-effects including cardiovascular disease, chronic fatigue, chronic pain, heightened pain perception, recurrent infections, poor healing, irritability, anxiety, depression as well as impaired concentration and memory. Severe sleep deprivation can lead to psychosis, confusion and in extreme cases, even death.

How much sleep do I need per night?
The duration of time needed for sleep changes as you age. Infants and adolescents need more sleep to fuel their growth. As you age you may find that you need less and less sleep. Rather than focus on the number of hours spent sleeping, you really should ask yourself if you feel well rested on awakening? If not, you did not get enough sleep. Although we progress through different phases of sleep during the night, it is the deepest stage of non-REM sleep where your body does most of its housekeeping. Recent research has found that the brain clears away waste products at night, which suggests that poor sleep may increase your risk of dementia (Xie, L. et. al 2014). Generally, most adults feel their best with an uninterrupted 7-9 hours of sleep.

How can I improve my sleep?
If you can improve your sleep, this is one of the best things you can do for your health. Do not get frustrated by the process. Instead, let it come naturally and keep it simple by trying these easy ideas. Remember, you need to train your body to sleep well.

Ideas for Sound Sleep

Sleep Hygiene	1. Develop a bedtime ritual.
	2. Avoid television/laptop/mobile screen time two hours prior to bed.
	3. Consider taking a warm, calming bath.
	4. Sleep in a cool and dark room away from noise and distractions.
	5. Get comfortable by using pillows to support body and wear non-restrictive pajamas.
Diet	1. Avoid caffeine, sugar. artificial sweeteners and flour as they can be stimulating.
	2. Limit fluid intake several hours before bedtime and empty your bladder prior to bed to minimize night-time bathroom trips.

Exercise	1. Exercise daily. 2. Do not exercise at night as it can keep you awake.
Home Remedies	1. Lavender essential oil (a few sprays under pillow or drop of oil on the upper lip) 2. Melatonin 3. Review the day with your loved one.

Resources:

1. "National Sleep Foundation - Sleep Research & Education." National Sleep Foundation - Sleep Research & Education. Web. 17 Jan. 2015. <http://sleepfoundation.org/>.
2. "Why Sleep Matters." Why Sleep Matters. Web. 18 Jan. 2015. <http://healthysleep.med.harvard.edu/healthy/matters>.
3. Xie, L., H. Kang, Q. Xu, M. J. Chen, Y. Liao, M. Thiyagarajan, J. O'donnell, D. J. Christensen, C. Nicholson, J. J. Iliff, T. Takano, R. Deane, and M. Nedergaard. "Sleep Drives Metabolite Clearance from the Adult Brain." Science 342.6156 (2013): 373-77. Print.

Chapter 7

The Unparalleled Compromise of Continuous Stress

What is stress?
Stress is a physiologic state of mental or emotional strain resulting from some form of adverse or demanding circumstance. Stress can be triggered by many things that are real or perceived and can be experienced in variable degrees in different individuals.

How can stress affect your health?
It is important to remember, that not all stress is bad. It is a natural physiologic response that can be life-saving in some situations such as escaping a burning building. During a stressful situation, your body releases particular compounds and hormones that heighten your senses, tense your muscles and increase your heart and lung function to get you ready to run. In short bursts it is a blessing; however, with chronic stress, the prolonged and continuous exposure of your body tissues to these compounds is detrimental to your health. The

With stress, perception is everything

stress response boosts certain organ systems such as your heart, lungs and muscles which are immediately needed for survival over others such as your immune, digestive and reproductive systems. As a result, their activity is limited and impaired. Once the threat has passed, these other body systems restore themselves. If they are unable to do so or if stress remains chronic, serious health problems can develop including stomach ulcers, heart disease, high blood pressure, diabetes, depression and anxiety and in rare cases, death.

What are common stress-related symptoms?
Everyone feels and responds to stress in different ways. Some individuals predominately experience digestive symptoms, whereas others may develop sleeplessness, headaches, depressed mood, anger or irritability. Because chronic stress can impair the immune system, there is an increased propensity for more frequent and severe infections, including the common cold or flu.

How can I decrease and better cope with stress in my life?
It is never too late to start taking steps towards maintaining your health and outlook which can reduce or prevent the ill-effects of chronic stress. Some tips include:

1. **Surround yourself with positive people** and those who can provide emotional and other support.
2. **Set priorities** and decide what must be get done first, what can wait and learn to say no to new tasks if they are putting an excess load on you.
3. **Review your accomplishments** at the end of the day and not what you have been unable to do.
4. **Limit your focus on problems**.
5. **Schedule healthy and relaxing activities** such as spending time with loved ones or doing your favorite hobby.
6. **Exercise regularly** as even just 20-30 minutes of mild-moderate exercise can help boost your mood.
7. **Explore stress relieving exercises** such as meditation, yoga, tai chi, or other movement activities.
8. **Seek help from a qualified mental health care provider** if you feel overwhelmed and cannot cope, have suicidal thoughts, or are using drugs or alcohol to artificially elevate your mood.

Marwa Ahmed MD, Andre Panagos MD

Resources:
1. "Fact Sheet on Stress." NIMH RSS. Web. 16 Jan. 2015. <http://www.nimh.nih.gov/health/publications/stress/index.shtml>.

Chapter 8

The Wonderful and Powerful Effect of Posture

The health of your spine is not independent of posture. In today's more cerebral society, most of us are employed for our brains and not our brawn. Unfortunately, most of these jobs come with the tragedy of a computer, desk and a chair. And so, we go to work and sit, and sit, then we go home and sit some more. You probably sit more than 10 hours every day. Not only is it impossible to have good posture while sitting for a prolonged period of time, but sitting also puts added pressure on your spinal discs, ligaments and nerves, which contribute to further wear-and-tear.

Why is good posture so important?
Good posture contributes to a range of health benefits. Good sitting and standing posture entails keeping your spine in optimal alignment with your ears over the shoulders and shoulders over your hips. When the bones of your spine are aligned properly, the weight of your head and torso are evenly distributed through the vertebral bones and discs which decreases their risk of injury. Also

the small and large muscles that support your spine are relaxed and ready to fire when you need to move. When you sit, you muscles constantly work hard and eventually fatigue, which research has demonstrated increases your risk of a back injury and chronic back pain.

What can I do to improve my posture?
You can improve your posture and decrease your risk of back pain and injury by doing some very simple activities.

1. ***Imagery.*** Think of a straight line passing through your body from the ceiling to the floor (your ears, shoulders, hips and knees should line up vertically). Now imagine that a strong cord attached to your breastbone is pulling your chest and rib cage upward, making you taller. Try to hold your pelvis level and don't allow the lower back to sway. Think of stretching your head toward the ceiling, increasing the space between your rib cage and pelvis. Picture yourself as a ballerina or ice skater rather than a soldier at attention.

2. ***Shoulder blade squeeze.*** Sit up straight in a chair with your hands resting on your thighs. Keep your shoulders down and your chin level. Slowly draw your shoulders back and squeeze your shoulder blades together. Hold for a count of five then relax. Repeat five times.

3. ***Upper-body stretch.*** Stand facing a corner with your arms raised, hands flat against the walls, elbows at shoulder height. Place one foot ahead of the other. Bending your forward knee, exhale as you lean your body toward the corner. Keep your back straight and your chest and head up. You should feel a stretch across the front of your chest. Hold this position for 20-30 seconds. Relax and repeat five times.

4. ***Arm-across-chest stretch.*** Raise your right arm to shoulder level in front of you and bend the arm at the elbow, keeping the forearm parallel to the floor. Grasp the right elbow with your left hand and gently pull it across your chest so that you feel a stretch in the right upper arm and shoulder. Hold for 20 seconds

then relax both arms. Repeat on the other side. Repeat five times on each side.

I do not have a lot of time to do exercise, what else can I do?
Trade in your standard sitting desk for an adjustable height standing desk. This gives you the opportunity to stand at your desk and increase your mobility during the day. Remember to break up your standing with periodic sitting breaks for lunch or meetings. If you have to sit at your desk, you can improve your comfort, work performance and reduce your risk of musculoskeletal injury with frequent 1-2 minute micro-breaks every 20-30 minutes or a 5 minute break every hour. Remember you cannot sit or stand all day long, so remember to take breaks throughout the day. The goal is to keep your muscles active as research has shown that prolonged sitting causes your muscles to lose their coordination and in severe cases can shut down the muscles all together. By keeping your muscles active throughout the day they are ready to support your activities and they also allow you to burn more calories keeping your weight under control as well.

Will poor posture during certain activities increase my risk of injury?
Activities that may result in injury when done with poor posture include weight training, carrying a heavy item or bag, which some have called, "poshitis"; using your mobile phone with your head hanging forward referred to as "text neck"; sitting with your legs crossed or slouching in your chair; and cradling the phone between your head and shoulder. It is important to think about your posture when doing these activities repeatedly or think of other ways to accomplish the task without using poor biomechanics such as a taking frequent breaks, using a standing desk mentioned previously or by asking for assistance.

Resources:
1. "Common Posture Mistakes and Fixes." - Live Well. Web. 01 Feb. 2015. <http://www.nhs.uk/Livewell/Backpain/Pages/back-pain-and-common-posture-mistakes.aspx>.
2. Nachemson, Alf L. "The Lumbar Spine An Orthopaedic Challenge." Spine 1.1 (1976): 59-71. Print.
3. "New Releases." 4 Ways to Turn Good Posture into Less Back Pain. Web. 18 Jan. 2015. <http://www.health.harvard.edu/healthbeat/4-ways-to-turn-

good-posture-into-less-back-pain>.
4. "Pilates and Back Pain - Part 1." Experience Pilates. 21 May 2012. Web. 18 Jan. 2015. <https://experiencepilates.wordpress.com/2012/05/21/pilates-and-back-pain-part-1/>.

Chapter 9

Jump-start Healing with Regenerative Medicine

What is regenerative medicine?

Your body is constantly focused on the repair, replacement and maintenance of tissues in your body. Tissues such as nerves, bone, tendon, muscle, ligament and connective tissue need constant maintenance to function properly. Long-standing disease, injury or poor lifestyle and dietary choices can overwhelm your body's natural repair mechanisms creating a cascade of breakdown. At first micro-injuries can occur which go unnoticed. Overtime repeat injury at the same location builds up resulting in a macro-injury that can be very noticeable when it interferes with your daily or recreational activities. This is the time you consider a physician's visit.

Conventional treatments such as corticosteroid injections decrease inflammation and pain but do not repair tissues. Physical therapy is helpful in improving biomechanics which changes with the onset of pain and tissue damage as your body finds ways to limit further injury and pain. Surgery can help repair severe injuries but it is focused on salvaging the remaining tissues. New regenerative treatments have been found to restart and promote the healing process giving tissues a second chance to return to normal. Different approaches are used, based on the type of tissue injury and can include a subcutaneous perineural injection series, nerve hydrodissection, fascial interrogation/barbotage, prolotherapy, platelet-rich plasma and stem-cell based therapies. These therapies are gaining popularity as emerging clinical experience and research validates their utility and superiority in tissue repair compared with conventional treatments.

What steps are involved in regenerative medicine techniques?
The first step in regenerating tissue is to correctly and accurately identify the source of the injury or pain. This can be a challenge as by the time the patient is seen in the office their body has accommodated to the pain resulting in biomechanical deterioration. Biomechanical deterioration places surrounding tissue at risk of injury as well.

The first step is a comprehensive history and physical examination by an experienced physician. This is often accompanied by dynamic musculoskeletal imaging or magnetic resonance imaging (MRI) to determine the status of the underlying tissues. A treatment plan is then decided upon based on review of all the data. Treatment can include:

1. **Subcutaneous perineural injection series** involve the use of micro-injections to treat the small nerves within the fascia that often endure chronic nerve compression due to poor posture or biomechanics.
2. **Nerve hydrodissection** is an ultrasound technique for nerve compression which is used to free compressed nerves from surrounding soft tissues. This allows the blood supply to the local nerve tissue to recover which decreases nerve sensitivity.
3. **Fascial interrogation/barbotage** is an ultrasound technique for soft tissue compression which is used to soften fascial tissues that have been under chronic strain.
4. **Prolotherapy** is traditionally used to strengthen ligaments and tendons using a sclerosing agent.
5. **Platelet-rich plasma** therapies entail isolation and concentration of platelets from your blood followed by placement at the site of injury. Platelets contain a large and concentrated amount

of growth factors that, when released, hone in on the damaged tissue and signal for the recruitment of stem cells to repair the region.

6. **Stem cell treatments** are used similarly but can be more robust and entail the isolation of stem cells directly from either bone marrow or fat. These treatments are a good option should an individual have insufficient success with simpler treatments and can offer superiority by beginning the process of tissue repair to promote long-term success.

How can I maximize the effect of regenerative treatments?

Healing is not independent of your biochemical and nutritional status. The more you can optimize your diet and nutritional status, the higher the likelihood of a great outcome. It is also important to maintain and improve your overall musculoskeletal strength and flexibility as well as optimize your sleep habits and decrease your stress levels. Finally, you should quit smoking, frequent alcohol consumption and any other substance abuse.

What else do I need to know about these treatments?

Regenerative treatments take patience and should not be considered a quick fix. When they are effective they are considered more permanent than conventional treatments. You have the best chance of having a great result with patience and some hard work on your part.

Resources:

1. Amable, Paola, Rosana Bizon Carias, Marcus Vinicius Teixeira, Ítalo Da Cruz Pacheco, Ronaldo José Corrêa Do Amaral, José Granjeiro, and Radovan Borojevic. "Platelet-rich Plasma Preparation for Regenerative Medicine: Optimization and Quantification of Cytokines and Growth Factors." Stem Cell Research & Therapy 4.3 (2013): 67. Print.
1. Dechellis, David M., and Megan Helen Cortazzo. "Regenerative Medicine in the Field of Pain Medicine: Prolotherapy, Platelet-rich Plasma Therapy, and Stem Cell Therapy—Theory and Evidence." Techniques in Regional Anesthesia and Pain Management 15.2 (2011): 74-80. Print.

About the Authors

Marwa Ahmed MD, MS, FAAPMR

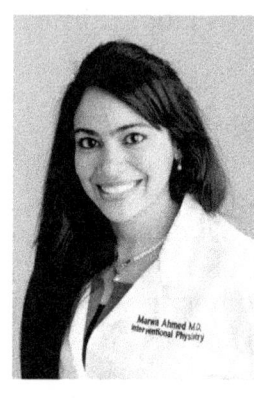

Dr. Marwa Ahmed specializes in sports, spine and musculoskeletal medicine which dovetail with her innate intrigue in human musculoskeletal anatomy and kinesiology. With a master of science degree in human genetics from the University of Michigan, Dr. Ahmed brings a unique and biological perspective to her practice. She has strong interests in regenerative medicine and nutritional genomics as well as their specific applications in the field of musculoskeletal medicine, including the molecular mechanisms that underlie physical performance, cellular aging, injury and repair. Dr. Ahmed's treatment philosophy is one that incorporates and optimizes an individual's nutritional status to cultivate and promote tissue healing as well as prevent injury. This approach has frequently and almost consistently lead to profound improvements in her patients' wide range of symptoms, injuries and illnesses.

Dr. Ahmed received her medical degree from the Weill Cornell Medical College in Qatar, where she was also peer selected as the recipient of the Good Physician Award. She completed her internship at the Virginia Commonwealth University Hospital and residency in Physical Medicine and Rehabilitation at New York Presbyterian Hospital – Columbia College of Physician and Surgeons and Weill Cornell Medical College. During residency, she also rotated at the Hospital for Special Surgery and Memorial-Sloan Kettering Cancer Center where she treated and managed patients with complex orthopedic injuries and cancer-related musculoskeletal complications. She is board-certified by the American Board of Physical Medicine and Rehabilitation as well as the American Board of Integrative and Holistic Medicine.

Dr. Ahmed is a member of several scientific organizations including the American Medical Society for Sports Medicine, American Academy of Physical Medicine and Rehabilitation, International Spine Intervention Society, and the New York County Medical Society.

Andre Panagos MD, MSc, FAAPMR

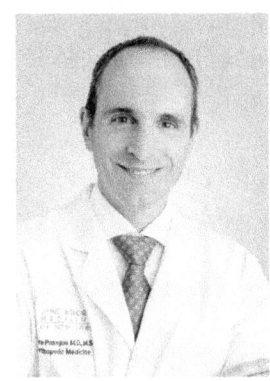

A true pioneer in regenerative spine and sports medicine, New York City physician Andre Panagos M.D. has been treating, preventing, and healing chronic pain for nearly two decades. His practice is dedicated to regenerative spine and sports medicine which makes Dr. Panagos a physician at the forefront of a new renaissance in medicine. He is board-certified by the American Board of Physical Medicine and Rehabilitation, with an additional board certification in pain medicine. He is also a New York State certified medical acupuncturist, a practitioner in functional medicine and regenerative medicine and has extensive training in interventional ultrasonography.

Dr. Panagos continuously reads medical texts and journals to further his education and travels throughout the country in order to learn and teach cutting edge techniques in his field. He believes in utilizing the most advanced practices and techniques to maximize function and improve quality of life, irrespective of often severe medical conditions. Dr. Panagos believes it is imperative to optimize health to allow the body to overcome disease. He has also been very fortunate and humbled to treat patients who were thought of as untreatable and return them to a fulfilling life, sometimes decades after the onset of serious illness.

Dr. Panagos is a fellow of the American Academy of Physical Medicine and Rehabilitation, and a member of several scientific organizations including the American Medical Society for Sports Medicine, North American Spine Society, International Spinal Intervention Society, Institute of Functional Medicine, American Institute of Ultrasound in Medicine, American Association of Orthopaedic Medicine and the New York County Medical Society. He is involved nationally with the American Academy of Physical Medicine and Rehabilitation and is a reviewer for the Archives of Physical Medicine and Rehabilitation and PM&R journals.

Dr. Panagos received his medical degree and Master of Science degrees from St. George's University, School of Medicine. He completed his internship and residency in Physical Medicine and Rehabilitation at the University of Washington, followed by a Sports and Interventional Spine Fellowship in the Department of Orthopedic Surgery at Beth Israel Medical Center. Dr. Panagos also trained in medical acupuncture at the Helms Medical Institute/UCLA and was educated at the Institute of Functional Medicine.

Dr. Panagos is currently a Clinical Assistant Professor in the Department of Rehabilitation Medicine at New York University Langone Medical Center. He previously served as an Assistant Attending Physiatrist at NewYork-Presbyterian Hospital and as an Assistant Professor in the Department of Rehabilitation Medicine at Weill Cornell Medical College. He was the founding co-director of The Spine Center at NewYork-Presbyterian Hospital and was the recipient of the first Willibald Nagler Clinical Scholar Award. Dr. Panagos was also honored with the

2009 Resident teaching award in the Department of Rehabilitation Medicine at Weill Cornell Medical College.

Dr. Panagos has been involved in medical education for many years, including research articles, textbook chapters, television and magazine interviews and has given many national and international lectures. Dr. Panagos released his textbook, Spine-A Rehabilitation Medicine Quick Reference, in 2010 which broadly covers the complex field of spine care and looks forward to releasing several more titles for his patients.